Mnemonics on Pathology and Microbiology

Mnemonics on Pathology and Microbiology

Krishna N Sharma
BPT MPT (Neuro) PhD (VC) CPTD (Ortho) D Ac MOPC
Academic Chairman
DLS Institute for Health and Wellness
Muhammadabad Gohana, Mau, Uttar Pradesh, India
Editor
The Scientific Research Journal of India
General Secretary
The Online Physio Community, India
Ex-HOD
Jeevan Jyoti Institute of Medical Sciences
Allahabad, Uttar Pradesh, India

JAYPEE BROTHERS MEDICAL PUBLISHERS (P) LTD
New Delhi • Panama City • London • Philadelphia (USA)

Jaypee Brothers Medical Publishers (P) Ltd

Headquarters
Jaypee Brothers Medical Publishers (P) Ltd
4838/24, Ansari Road, Daryaganj
New Delhi 110 002, India
Phone: +91-11-43574357
Fax: +91-11-43574314
Email: jaypee@jaypeebrothers.com

Overseas Offices

J.P. Medical Ltd
83 Victoria Street, London
SW1H 0HW (UK)
Phone: +44-2031708910
Fax: +02-03-0086180
Email: info@jpmedpub.com

Jaypee-Highlights Medical Publishers Inc.
City of Knowledge, Bld. 237, Clayton
Panama City, Panama
Phone: + 507-301-0496
Fax: + 507-301-0499
Email: cservice@jphmedical.com

Jaypee Brothers Medical Publishers (P) Ltd
17/1-B Babar Road, Block-B, Shaymali
Mohammadpur, Dhaka-1207
Bangladesh
Mobile: +08801912003485
Email: jaypeedhaka@gmail.com

Jaypee Brothers Medical Publishers (P) Ltd
Shorakhute, Kathmandu
Nepal
Phone: +00977-9841528578
Email: jaypee.nepal@gmail.com

Website: www.jaypeebrothers.com
Website: www.jaypeedigital.com

Inquiries for bulk sales may be solicited at: jaypee@jaypeebrothers.com

Mnemonics on Pathology and Microbiology

First Edition: **2013**

ISBN: 978-93-5090-297-4

Printed at: S. Narayan & Sons

Dedicated to

My Parents

Dr L Sharma
and
Smt Chintamani Sharma

Preface

The term mnemonic came from name of the Greek Goddess of memory—*Mnemosyne*, the mother of the Muses whose name means 'remembrance'. The mnemonics had always been a very easy, interesting and effective tool for learning. These memory pearls make the learning enjoyable. During the studies, I had been passionate about making the mnemonics. This passion resulted into a good list of self-made mnemonics which is in your hand right now.

I hope you will find this to be a useful book that facilitates the speed of memorizing the lengthy material. Hope you will appreciate this and send your comments and suggestions to me.

Krishna N Sharma
Email: *dr.krisharma@gmail.com*
Web: *http://www.krishna.info.ms*

Acknowledgments

First and foremost, I would like to thank my family for their constant support. I also thank the cosmic energies for their kind guidance.

I would like to acknowledge the guidance of Shri Jitendar P Vij (Group Chairman), Mr Ankit Vij (Managing Director), Mr Tarun Duneja (Director-Publishing) and Ms Samina Khan (PA to Director-Publishing) of M/s Jaypee Brothers Medical Publishers (P) Ltd, New Delhi, India, who made it possible to make this text more efficient.

I would like to thank all my friends and colleagues for their support and advice.

Contents

1. Alimentary System 1
Colon Carcinoma: Etiology 1
Carcinoid Syndrome: Components 1
Colon Cancer: Risk Factors 2
Escherichia coli: Major Subtypes and Key Point of Each 2
Food Poisoning: Bugs Inducing 3
Kwashiorkor: Distinguishing from Marasmus 4
Nematodes: Ones Spreading by Egg Ingestion 4
Oral Cancer Risks 5
Peptic Ulcer: Associated Causative Factors 5
Pancreatitis: Drugs Causing it 6
Ulcerative Colitis: Features 6

2. Cardiovascular System 8
Atherosclerosis: Risk Factors 8
Aneurysm: Types 9

Buerger's Disease: Features 9
Cardiovascular Risk Factors 10
Deep Venous Thrombosis: Diagnosis 11
Deep Venous Thrombosis: Genetic Causes 11
Endocarditis: Laboratory Results Suggesting it 12
Endocarditis: Causes of Culture Negative Endocarditis 12
Endocarditis: Indications for Surgery 13
Fat Embolism: Findings 14
Hypertension: Secondary Hypertension (Causes) 14
Hemolytic Anemia: Types 15
Heart Failure: Causes 15
Kawasaki Disease: Diagnostic Criteria 16
Macrocytic Anemia: Differential 17
Myocardial Infarction: Complications 17
Myocardial Infarction: Sequence of Elevated Enzymes After MI 18
Protein S and Protein C: Function 19

Pericarditis: Findings 19
Thrombus: Possible Fates 19
Thrombotic Thrombocytopenic Purpura: Signs 20
Thrombotic Thrombocytopenic Purpura: Clinical Features 20
Virchow's Triad 21
Von Hippel-Lindau: Signs and Symptoms 21

3. Endocrine System 22
Addison's Disease: Features 22
Cushing Syndrome 23
Goiter: Differential 23
Hypothyroidism/Thyroiditis: Manifestations and Morphology 24
Hypercalcemia: Symptoms of Elevated Serum Levels 25
MEN I (Multiple Endocrine Neoplasia I) Syndrome: Components 25
MEN III (Multiple Endocrine Neoplasia III) Syndrome: Components 26

Pheochromocytoma: Three Most Common Symptoms 26
Pheochromocytoma: Common Symptoms 26
Thyroid Storm: Characteristics 27
Thyrotoxicosis Syndrome: Signs and Symptoms 27
Thyroid Carcinoma: Frequency (From Least Aggressive to Most Aggressive) 28

4. Integumentary System 29
Baldness Risk Factors 29
Leprosy: Early Signs (Diagnostic Criteria) 29
Pseudomonas aeruginosa: Features 30

5. Urinary System 31
Acute Post-streptococcal Glomerulonephritis: Classic Presentation 31
Calculi: Types 31
Gout: Factors that can Precipitate an Attack of Acute Gouty Arthritis 32
Hematuria: Urethral Causes 32

Hypokalemia: Clinical Features 33
Nephrotic Syndrome: Hallmark Findings 33
Nephritic Syndrome: Glomerular Diseases Commonly Presenting as Nephritic Syndrome 34
Renal Failure: Causes 35
Renal Failure (Chronic): Consequences 35
Urinary Tract Infection: Causing Microorganisms 37

6. Lymphatic System 38
AIDS Pathogens (T-cell Suppression) 38
Catalase Positive Organisms 39
Endotoxin: Features 39
Hypersplenism: Criteria 40
IgA Protease-Producing Bacteria 40
Macrocytosis: Non-B_{12}/Folate Causes 41
Microcytic Anemia: Causes 41
Picorna Viridae: Members 42
Symptoms of TTP/HUS 42
Sarcoidosis: Summarized 43

Vaccines: Types 44
Wiskott-Aldrich Syndrome: Symptom Triad 44

7. Muscular System 45
McArdle's Syndrome 45
Tetanus: Treatment for Infection 46

8. Nervous System 47
Alzheimer's Disease: Features 47
Dandy-Walker Syndrome: Components 47
Meningitis: Risk Factors 48
Meningitis: Most Common Organisms 48
Neuroblastoma: Features 49
Parkinsonism: Essential Features 49
Pyogenic Meningitis: Likeliest Bug in Age Group (in Order from Death to Birth) 50
Tabes Dorsalis: Morphology 50
Toxoplasma gondii: Manifestations 51
Wernicke-Korsakoff's Psychosis: Findings 51

9. Pulmonary System 53

Adult Respiratory Distress Syndrome: Causes 53

Bronchial Obstruction: Consequences 54

Interstitial Lung Disease: Causes 54

Influenza Infection: Clinical Manifestations 55

Klebsiella: Details 56

Pulmonary Embolism: Risk Factors 56

Pulmonary Fibrosis: Differential of Both Upper and Lower Lobes 57

Pneumothorax: Presentation 58

Respiratory Distress Syndrome in Infants: Major Risk Factors 58

10. Reproductive System 59

Endometrial Carcinoma: Risk Factors 59

Gynecomastia: Causes 60

Ovarian Cancers: Important Types by WHO Classification 60

Polycystic Ovarian Disease: Clinical Features 61

Scrotum Masses 62

11. Skeletal System.. 63
Carcinomas Having Tendency to Metastasize to Bone 63
Marble Bone Disease: Signs and Symptoms 63
Osteomyelitis: Complications 64
Rheumatoid Arthritis: Features 64

12. Miscellaneous.. 66
Capsulated Bacteria 66
Common Cold: Viral Causes 67
Fragile-X Syndrome: Features 67
Necrosis: The Four Types 68
RNA Viruses: Negative Stranded 68
RNA Viruses: Positive Stranded 69
RNA Enveloped Viruses 69
Staphylococcus aureus: Diseases Caused 70
Streptococcus pyogenes: Diseases Caused 71
Streptococcus pyogenes: Virulence Factors 71
Turner Syndrome: Components 72
Urease: Positive Organisms 72
Whipple's Disease: Full Features 73

Index 75

CHAPTER

1

Alimentary System

COLON CARCINOMA: ETIOLOGY

SCRAP

- **S**trong family history of colon cancer
- **C**hronic ulcerative colitis
- **R**atio of animal fat:fiber diet
- **A**denomatous polyps
- **P**olyposis (familial).

CARCINOID SYNDROME: COMPONENTS

Cut CARD

- **Cut**aneous flushing
- **C**ramping

- **A**sthmatic wheezing
- **R**ight sided valvular heart lesions
- **D**iarrhea.

COLON CANCER: RISK FACTORS

LAHU

- **L**ow fiber, high fat diet
- **A**denomatous polyps
- **H**eridity
- **U**lcerative colitis.

ESCHERICHIA COLI: MAJOR SUBTYPES AND KEY POINT OF EACH

Enter and HIT

Enterohemorrhagic:

- **H**US from hamburgers

Enteroinvasive:

- **I**mmune-mediated inflammation

Enterotoxigenic:

- **T**raveller's diarrhea.

FOOD POISONING: BUGS INDUCING

Contaminated Stuff Eater Can Start Vomiting Very Badly

- ***C**lostridium botulinum* (canned foods)
- ***S**almonella* (poultry, meat, eggs)
- ***E**scherichia coli* O157-H7 (undercooked meat, especially hamburgers)
- ***C**lostridium perfringens* (reheated meat)
- ***S**taphylococcus aureus* (meats, mayo, custard)
- ***V**ibrio parahaemolyticus* (seafood)
- ***V**ibrio vulnificus* (seafood)
- ***B**acillus cereus* (reheated rice).

KWASHIORKOR: DISTINGUISHING FROM MARASMUS

FAME

- **F**atty liver
- **A**nemia
- **M**alabsorption
- **E**dema.

NEMATODES: ONES SPREADING BY EGG INGESTION

AT Egg

- ***A**scaris lumbricoides*
- ***T**richuris trichiura*
- ***E**nterobius vermicularis.*

ORAL CANCER RISKS

BATH PAL

- **B**ad oral hygiene
- **A**lcohol
- **T**obacco
- **H**uman papilloma virus
- **P**lummer-Vinson syndrome
- **A**sbestos
- **L**eukoplakia.

PEPTIC ULCER: ASSOCIATED CAUSATIVE FACTORS

HAZAM Sab

- **H**ypercalcemia
- **A**spirin
- **Z**ollinger-Ellison
- **A**cidity
- **M**ultiple endocrine neoplasia (MEN) type I
- **S**moking.

PANCREATITIS: DRUGS CAUSING IT

FAT SEES PEN

- **F**urosemide
- **A**ngiotensin-converting enzyme (ACF) inhibitors
- **T**hiazides
- **S**teroids
- **E**thacrynic acid
- **E**rythromycin
- **S**ulfas
- **P**enicillamine
- **E**strogen
- **N**onsteroidal anti-inflammatory drugs (NSAIDs).

ULCERATIVE COLITIS: FEATURES

LUSt CREATION

- **L**arge intestine
- **U**lcers

- **S**tools bloody
- **C**arcinoma (risk)
- **R**emnants of old ulcers (pseudopolyps)
- **E**xtraintestinal manifestations
- **A**bscesses in crypts
- **T**oxic megacolon (risk)
- **I**nflamed, red, granular mucosa
- **O**riginates at rectum
- **N**eutrophil invasion.

Cardiovascular System

CHAPTER

2

ATHEROSCLEROSIS: RISK FACTORS

THE MATHS DID

- **T**riglycerdides and fats
- **H**ypertension
- **E**levated cholesterol
- **M**ale
- **A**ge
- **T**obacco
- **H**istory (family)
- **S**moking

- **D**iabetes mellitus
- **I**nactivity
- **D**iet/Drink.

ANEURYSM: TYPES

SAM reads ABCD

- **S**yphilitic
- **A**therosclerotic
- **M**ycotic
- **A**rteriovenous fistula
- **B**erry
- **C**apillary microaneurysm
- **D**issecting.

BUERGER'S DISEASE: FEATURES

GRIP PICS

- **G**angrene
- **R**aynaud's phenomenon

- **I**ntermittent claudication
- **P**ain, even at rest
- **P**hlebitis (superficial nodular)
- **I**diopathic
- **C**hronic ulceration
- **S**egmenting, thrombosing vasculitis.

CARDIOVASCULAR RISK FACTORS

BOSS Has FAILED

- **B**lood pressure
- **O**besity
- **S**moking
- **S**ex
- **H**omocystinemia
- **F**amily history
- **A**ge
- **I**nflammation (raised CRP)/Increased thrombosis
- **L**ipids

- **E**xercise
- **D**iabetes mellitus.

DEEP VENOUS THROMBOSIS: DIAGNOSIS

3DVT

- **D**ilated superficial veins
- **D**iscoloration
- **D**oppler ultrasound
- **V**enography
- **T**enderness of calf and thigh.

DEEP VENOUS THROMBOSIS: GENETIC CAUSES

SACALA

- **S**-protein deficiency
- **A**ntithrombin III
- **C**-protein deficiency
- **A**PC (Activated protein C)

- Leiden (Factor V)
- Antiphospholipid antibody.

ENDOCARDITIS: LABORATORY RESULTS SUGGESTING IT

THe PEARL

- **T**hrombocytopenia
- **H**ematuria
- **P**roteinuria
- **E**levated erythrocyte sedimentation rate (ESR)
- **A**nemia
- **R**ed blood cell casta
- **L**eukocytosis, leukocytopenia.

ENDOCARDITIS: CAUSES OF CULTURE NEGATIVE ENDOCARDITIS

MISS NATO

- **M**ural endocarditis
- **I**nfection (Fungal)

- Slow growing fastidious organisms
- Subacute right-sided endocarditis
- Noninfectious endocarditis
- Antibiotic used previously
- Timing (cultures drawn at end of chronic course)
- Obligate intracellular organisms.

ENDOCARDITIS: INDICATIONS FOR SURGERY

PRIDE SIR

- **P**rosthetic valve endocarditis (most cases)
- **R**esection of mycotic aneurysm
- **I**neffective antimicrobial therapy (e.g. virus, fungi)
- **D**amaged valve (significant)
- **E**mbolization (repeated systemic)
- **S**upporative local complications with conduction abnormalities

- **I**nfection uncontrolled
- **R**efractory congestive heart failure.

FAT EMBOLISM: FINDINGS

He FUSed Bulb

- **H**istory of fracture
- **F**at in **U**rine/**S**putum
- **B**at-wing lung X-ray.

HYPERTENSION: SECONDARY HYPERTENSION (CAUSES)

CASH Payment

- **C**ushing's syndrome
- **A**orta coarctation
- **S**tenosis of renal arteries
- **H**yperaldosteronism
- **P**heochromocytoma.

HEMOLYTIC ANEMIA: TYPES

PEER SHIT

- **P**aroxysmal nocturnal hemoglobinuria
- **E**nzyme deficiencies: (G6P, pyruvate kinase)
- **E**rythroblastosis fetalis
- **R**ed blood cells (RBCs) trauma
- **S**ickle cell
- **H**ereditary sperocytosis
- **I**mmunohemolytics: (warm Ab, cold Ag)
- **T**halassemias: (alpha, beta).

HEART FAILURE CAUSES

I MADE HEART

- **I**nfection
- **M**yocardial infarct
- **A**rrhythmia
- **D**iet and lifestyle

- **E**ndocarditis
- **H**ypertension
- **E**mbolism
- **A**nemia
- **R**heumatic heart disease
- **T**hyrotoxicosis.

KAWASAKI DISEASE: DIAGNOSTIC CRITERIA

5 FIVE LCD

- **5** letters = 5 days, > 5 years old
- **F**ever > 5 days
- **I**diopathic polymorphic rash
- **V**asculitis
- **E**rythema of palms, soles (red palms, soles)
- **L**ymphoadenopathy (cervical)
- **C**onjunctivitis (bilateral)
- **D**ryness of (a) lips and month (b) palms and soles.

MACROCYTIC ANEMIA: DIFFERENTIAL

PART B and C

- **P**regnancy
- **A**lcohol
- **R**eticulocytosis
- **T**hyroid disease (i.e. hypothyroidism)
- **B**$_{12}$ and folate deficiency
- **C**irrhosis and chronic liver disease.

MYOCARDIAL INFARCTION: COMPLICATIONS

RAPID CAT

- **R**upture (septum, ventricle, papillary muscle)
- **A**neurysm (ventricle)
- **P**ericarditis
- **I**nfarctions
- **D**ressler's syndrome/Death
- **C**ongestive cardiac failure
- **A**rrhythmias (SVT, VT, VF)
- **T**amponade/Thromboembolic disorders.

MYOCARDIAL INFARCTION: COMPLICATIONS

PIA MEAL

- **P**ericarditis
- **I**nfarction progressive
- **A**rrhythmia
- **M**yocardial rupture
- **E**mbolism (systemic)
- **A**neurysm (ventricular)
- **L**eft ventricular failure (LVF)

MYOCARDIAL INFARCTION: SEQUENCE OF ELEVATED ENZYMES AFTER MI

The CALI

- **T**roponin
- **C**reatine kinase-MB isoenzyme (CK-MB)
- **A**spartate transaminase (AST)
- **L**actate dehydrogenase (LDH 1).

PROTEIN S AND PROTEIN C: FUNCTION

Stop Coagulation

- The function of these proteins is to inhibit coagulation.

PERICARDITIS: FINDINGS

RICE Plate

- **R**ub
- **I**ncreased jugular venous pressure (JVP)
- **C**hest pain
- **E**lectrocardiographic (ECG) changes
- **P**ulsus paradoxus.

THROMBUS: POSSIBLE FATES

DO People Earn

- **D**issolution
- **O**rganization and repair

- **P**ropagation
- **E**mbolization.

THROMBOTIC THROMBOCYTOPENIC PURPURA: SIGNS

RAT on FaN

- **R**enal problems
- **A**nemia
- **T**hrombocytopenia
- **F**ever
- **N**eurologic dysfunction.

THROMBOTIC THROMBOCYTOPENIC PURPURA: CLINICAL FEATURES

NEw PART

- **N**eurological deficits
- **E**mergency room (ER) admission (as it is an emergency)
- **P**latelet count low
- **A**nemia (microangiopathic hemolytic)

- **R**enal failure
- **T**emperature rise.

VIRCHOW'S TRIAD

VIB

- **V**ascular trauma
- **I**ncreased coagulability.
- **B**lood flow reduced (stasis).

VON HIPPEL-LINDAU: SIGNS AND SYMPTOMS

Please Know HIPPEL

- Pancreas
- Kidney cysts
- **H**emanigoblastomas
- **I**ncreased renal cancer
- **P**heochromocytoma
- **P**ort-wine stains
- **E**ye dysfunction
- **L**iver.

CHAPTER 3

Endocrine System

ADDISON'S DISEASE: FEATURES

MAD SHIN

- **M**eningcoccus disseminated intravascular coagulation (DIC)
- **A**utoimmune
- **D**estruction by cancer, infection, vascular insufficiency
- **S**arcoidosis, granulomatous such as tuberculosis (TB) histiomycosis
- **H**ypotension/Hyponatremia
- **I**atrogenic
- **N**elson's syndrome (postadrenalectomy, increased adrenocorticotropic hormone).

CUSHING SYNDROME

Hey$_{(4)}$ Can$_{(4)}$ U SING$_{(2,1,1,2)}$

- **H**ypercortisolism/**H**yperglycemia/**H**ypertension/**H**irsutism
- **C**ollagen fiber weakness/**C**entral obesity/**C**ervical fat pads/ **C**omedones (acne)
- **U**rinary free corisol and glucose increase
- **S**triae/**S**uppressed immunity
- **I**atrogenic (Increased administration of corticosteroids)
- **N**oniatrogenic neoplasms
- **G**lucose intolerance/**G**rowth retardation.

GOITER: DIFFERENTIAL

Oh! TIGER

- **O**nset of puberty
- **T**hyrotoxicosis/**T**umor/**T**hyroiditis (Hashimoto's)

- **I**odine deficiency
- **G**oitrogens
- **E**nzyme deficiencies
- **R**eproduction (pregnancy).

HYPOTHYROIDISM/THYROIDITIS: MANIFESTATIONS AND MORPHOLOGY

CHASMIS

- **C**retinism/**C**onstipation/**C**old intolerance
- **H**ashimoto's disease
- **A**ddison disease
- **S**ubacute thyroiditis
- **M**yxedema coma
- **I**nfectious-subacute thyroiditis
- **S**ilent thyroiditis.

HYPERCALCEMIA: SYMPTOMS OF ELEVATED SERUM LEVELS

POSt

- **P**ain
- **O**vertone psychologically
- **S**tones (renal).

MEN I (MULTIPLE ENDOCRINE NEOPLASIA I) SYNDROME: COMPONENTS

PIPAT

- **P**ituatary
- **I**slets (pancreatic)
- **P**arathyroid
- **A**drenal cortex
- **T**hyroid, associated with peptic ulceration.

MEN III (MULTIPLE ENDOCRINE NEOPLASIA III) SYNDROME: COMPONENTS

MAN

- **M**edullary thyroid carcinoma
- **A**drenal of medulla (pheochromocytoma)
- **N**euroma (mucosal).

PHEOCHROMOCYTOMA: THREE MOST COMMON SYMPTOMS

Pheochromocytoma Has Diagnosis

- **P**alpitations
- **H**eadache
- **D**iaphoresis.

PHEOCHROMOCYTOMA: COMMON SYMPTOMS

PAPPU

- **P**aroxysmal rise in blood pressure (BP)
- **A**bdominal pain

- **P**alpitations
- **P**erspiration
- **U**rine pleomorphic microvilli (PMV) finding.

THYROID STORM: CHARACTERISTICS

SHIT

- **S**urgery
- **H**yperthyroidism
- **I**nfection or illness at childbirth
- **T**rauma.

THYROTOXICOSIS SYNDROME: SIGNS AND SYMPTOMS

FAME'S WEIGHT

- **F**atigability
- **A**nxiety
- **M**uscular weakness/Menstrual changes
- **E**motional lability
- **S**weating

- **W**eight loss with good appetite
- **E**ye changes
- **I**ncreased pulse rate
- **G**oiter
- **H**eat intolerance
- **T**remor.

THYROID CARCINOMA: FREQUENCY (FROM LEAST AGGRESSIVE TO MOST AGGRESSIVE)

People Find Me Atheist

- **P**apillary carcinoma
- **F**ollicular carcinoma
- **M**edullary thyroid carcinoma
- **A**naplastic carcinoma.

CHAPTER

4

Integumentary System

BALDNESS RISK FACTORS

Dangerous Don's Dear Hair Is Gone

- **D**iet
- **D**isease
- **D**rugs
- **H**ormones
- **I**njury to the scalp
- **G**enes.

LEPROSY: EARLY SIGNS (DIAGNOSTIC CRITERIA)

MAPS

- *Mycobacterium leprae* positive identification of under microscope

- **A**ffected superficial nerves enlarged and tender
- **P**aralysis.
- **S**ensory loss in affected skin.

PSEUDOMONAS AERUGINOSA: FEATURES

ISHA AERO-GUN

- **I**ron-containing lesions
- **S**lime capsule sometimes (in cardiac failure patient)
- **H**urt (injuries, burns)
- **A**dherin pili
- **A**erobic
- **E**xotoxin A
- **R**od/Resistance
- **O**dor of grapes
- **G**reen-blue dressings
- **U**rinary tract infections (UTIs)
- **N**egative gram.

Urinary System

CHAPTER

5

ACUTE POST-STREPTOCOCCAL GLOMERU-LONEPHRITIS: CLASSIC PRESENTATION

BSC

- **B**loated face (facial edema)
- **S**ore throat: 1 week ago
- **C**oke-colored urine.

CALCULI: TYPES

CACU

- **C**alcium
- **A**mmonium magnesium phosphate
- **C**ystine
- **U**ric acid.

GOUT: FACTORS THAT CAN PRECIPITATE AN ATTACK OF ACUTE GOUTY ARTHRITIS

DANNI

- **D**iuretics
- **A**lcohol
- **N**ight attacks
- **N**ephronal disease
- **I**njury.

HEMATURIA: URETHRAL CAUSES

STUN

- **S**tone
- **T**umor
- **U**rethritis
- **N**eoplasm.

HYPOKALEMIA: CLINICAL FEATURES

WITCH Has PAD Protection

- **W**eakness of muscles
- **I**ncreases P-R interval, T wave and prominent U wave
- **T**etany
- **C**ramps
- **H**epatic encephalopathy (chances)
- **H**ypotonia
- **P**olyuria
- **A**rrhythmias
- **D**igoxin toxicity
- **P**aralytic ileus increases.

NEPHROTIC SYNDROME: HALLMARK FINDINGS

PLACE

- **P**roteinuria
- **L**ipid up

- **A**lbumin down
- **C**holesterol up
- **E**dema.

NEPHRITIC SYNDROME: GLOMERULAR DISEASES COMMONLY PRESENTING AS NEPHRITIC SYNDROME

Miss Gaga Is Singing RAP

- **M**embranoproliferative
- **G**oodpasture's
- **I**gA nephropathy
- **S**ystemic lupus erythematosus (SLE)
- **R**apidly progressive glomerulonephritis (RGPN)
- **A**lport's
- **P**ost-streptococcal.

RENAL FAILURE: CAUSES

A Glance on The Very Important Urinary Disease

- **A**cute tubular necrosis
- **G**lomerular disease
- **T**ubulointerstitial nephritis
- **V**ascular obstruction
- **I**nfection
- **U**rinary obstruction
- **D**iffuse intravascular coagulation.

RENAL FAILURE (CHRONIC): CONSEQUENCES

Everybody SHow Me Various Or One PACH on HIP

Anemia

- **E**rythropoietin (EPO) is less

Electrolyte imbalance

- **S**odium loss/gain
- **H**yperkalemia
- **M**etabolic acidosis

Bone alterations

- **V**on Recklinghausen
- **O**steomalacia
- **O**steoporosis

Cardiopulmonary

- **P**ericarditis
- **A**therosclerosis
- **C**ongestive heart failure (CHF)
- **H**ypertension

Gastrointestinal (GI) disturbances

- **H**emorrhagic gastritis
- **I**ntractable hiccups
- **P**eptic ulcer disease.

URINARY TRACT INFECTION: CAUSING MICROORGANISMS

SEEKS PEP

- ***S****taphylococcus saprophyticus*
- ***E****nterococcus faecalis*
- ***E****nterobacter cloacae*
- ***K****lebsiella*
- ***S****erratia marcescens*
- ***P****seudomonas aeroginosa*
- ***E****scherichia coli*
- ***P****roteus mirabilis*

CHAPTER

Lymphatic System 6

AIDS PATHOGENS (T-CELL SUPPRESSION)

The Pathogens May Cause Complete T-Cell Collapse

- *Toxoplasma gondii*
- *Pneumocystis carinii*
- *Mycobacterium avium intracellulare*
- Cytomegalovirus (CMV)
- *Cryptococcus neoformans*
- Tuberculosis
- *Cryptosporidium parvum*
- *Candida albicans*

CATALASE POSITIVE ORGANISMS

SCAPE

- ***S**taphylococcus aureus*
- ***C**andida*
- ***A**spergillus*
- ***P**seudomonas*
- ***E**nterobacter*.

ENDOTOXIN FEATURES

NO! I DON'T NEED Her

- **N**eutrophil chemotaxis
- **O**-antigen
- **I**nterleukin-1 (IL-1)
- **D**isseminated intravascular coagulation (DIC)
- **O**uter membrane
- **N**itric oxide
- **T**umor necrosis factor (TNF)

- **N**egative (gram-bacteria)
- **E**ndothelial cells
- **E**dema
- **D**eath
- **H**eat stable.

HYPERSPLENISM: CRITERIA

Cant Remember Hyper Splenism

- **C**ytopenias
- **R**esponse to splenectomy
- **H**ypercellular or normal marrow
- Splenomegaly.

IgA PROTEASE-PRODUCING BACTERIA

Not So Handsome

- *Neisseria*
- *Streptococcus pneumoniae*
- *Haemophilus influenzae.*

MACROCYTOSIS: NON-B_{12}/FOLATE CAUSES

PALER HAND

- **P**regnancy
- **A**lcohol
- **L**iver disease
- **E**ndocrine (hypothyroidism)
- **R**eticulocytes
- **H**emolysis (especially chronic)
- **A**gglutination
- **N**eoplasia (including myelodysplasia)
- **D**rugs (especially myelosuppressives like chemotherapy, anti-HIV medicines).

MICROCYTIC ANEMIA: CAUSES

ITS

- **I**ron deficiency
- **T**halassemia
- **S**ideroblastic.

PICORNA VIRIDAE: MEMBERS

PREECH

- **P**oliovirus
- **R**hinovirus
- **E**chovirus
- **E**nterovirus
- **C**oronavirus
- **H**epatitis A.

SYMPTOMS OF TTP/HUS

My Favorite Teacher Never Roar

- **M**icroangiopathic hemolytic anemia
- **F**ever
- **T**hrombocytopenia
- **N**eurological symptoms
- **R**enal failure.

SARCOIDOSIS: SUMMARIZED

SARCOIDOSIS CLEARED

- **S**chaumann calcifications
- **A**steroid bodies (ACE) increase
- **R**enal calculi
- **C**D4 helper cells
- **O**cular lesions
- **I**mmune mediated noncaseating granulomas
- **D**iabetes insipidus
- **O**steopathy
- **S**kin (Subcutaneous nodules, erythema nodosum)
- **I**nterstitial lung fibrosis
- **S**eventh cranial nerves (CN) palsy
- **C**ardiomyopathy (restrictive)
- **L**ung disease
- **E**levated calcium level in serum and urine
- **A**nergy
- **R**espiratory complications

- **E**levated vitamin D value
- **D**yspnea.

VACCINES: TYPES

TRILS

- **T**oxoid
- **R**ecombinant
- **I**nactivated
- **L**ive
- **S**ubunit.

WISKOTT-ALDRICH SYNDROME: SYMPTOM TRIAD

SET

- **S**taphlococcal infections (Recurrent)
- **E**czema
- **T**hrombocytopenia.

CHAPTER

7

Muscular System

McARDLE'S SYNDROME

SELL My CARD

- **S**keletal muscle only
- **E**levated creatine kinase
- **L**actate levels fail to rise
- **M**yoglobinuria
- **C**ramping after exercise
- **A**ccumulated glycogen
- **R**ecessive inheritance
- **D**eficiency of muscle phosphorylase.

TETANUS: TREATMENT FOR INFECTION

SAD ART

- **S**edation
- **A**ntitoxin
- **D**ebridement
- **A**ntibiotic
- **R**elaxant
- **T**racheostomy.

CHAPTER

8 Nervous System

ALZHEIMER'S DISEASE: FEATURES

CALL DON

- **C**erebral cortex atrophy (diffuse)
- **A**ch reduction
- **L**anguage impairment
- **L**iving with dementia (MC in elderly)
- **D**own's syndrome
- **O**ld age
- **N**eurofibrillary tangles.

DANDY-WALKER SYNDROME: COMPONENTS

Warning For Vicky

- **W**ater on the brain
- **F**ourth (IV) ventricle dilated
- **V**ermis small.

MENINGITIS: RISK FACTORS

HE IS Chief Of SPAIN

- **H**ead trauma
- **E**xtreme age
- **I**mmunocompromised state
- **S**inusitis
- **C**ancer
- **O**titis
- **S**plenectomy
- **P**arameningeal infection
- **A**lcoholism
- **I**nfections (systemic, especially respiratory)
- **N**eurosurgical procedures.

MENINGITIS: MOST COMMON ORGANISMS

SIN

- *Streptococcus pneumoniae*
- *Influenzae (Haemophilus)*
- *Neisseria meningitidis.*

NEUROBLASTOMA: FEATURES

MY Clinical Neuroblastome

- **M**alignant
- **Y**oung
- **C**atecholamine secreting
- **N**uclei have “double minutes”.

PARKINSONISM: ESSENTIAL FEATURES

SMART

- **S**tooped posture
- **M**ask like face
- **A**kinesia
- **R**igidity
- **T**remor (resting).

PYOGENIC MENINGITIS: LIKELIEST BUG IN AGE GROUP (In order from death to birth)

She Never Had Entertainment

- ***S****treptococcus pneumoniae* (old folks)
- ***N****eisseria meningitis* (young adults)
- ***H****aemophilus influenzae* (older infants, kids)
- **E**scherichia coli (infants).

TABES DORSALIS: MORPHOLOGY

SAD SCRAP

- **S**yphilis
- **A**taxia
- **D**orsal column degeneration
- **S**hooting pain
- **C**harcot joints
- **R**eflexes decreased (deep tendon)
- **A**rgyll-Robertson pupils
- **P**roprioception impaired.

TOXOPLASMA GONDII: MANIFESTATIONS

MICE

- **M**yocarditis
- **I**llness like mononucleosis
- **C**horioretinitis/Congenital infection
- **E**ncephalitis.

WERNICKE-KORSAKOFF'S PSYCHOSIS: FINDINGS

CAT On RACK

Wernicke's encephalopathy (acute phase):

- **C**onfusion
- **A**taxia
- **T**hiamine tx.
- **O**phthalmoplegia

Korsakoff's psychosis (chronic phase):

- **R**etrograde amnesia
- **A**nterograde amnesia
- **C**onfabulation
- **K**orsakoff's psychosis.

Pulmonary System

CHAPTER 9

ADULT RESPIRATORY DISTRESS SYNDROME: CAUSES

DAD'S ADDRESS

- **D**rugs
- **A**spiration
- **D**IC
- **S**moke inhalation
- **A**cute pancreatitis
- **D**rowning
- **D**iffuse lung infection
- **R**adiation
- **E**mbolism
- **S**hock
- **S**epsis.

BRONCHIAL OBSTRUCTION: CONSEQUENCES

PLEase Play ABBA

- **P**leural adhesions
- **L**ipid pneumonia
- **E**mphysema
- **P**leuritis
- **A**telectasis
- **B**ronchiectasis
- **B**roncho and lobar pneumonia
- **A**bscess.

INTERSTITIAL LUNG DISEASE: CAUSES

DISCO AIR

- **D**rugs
- **I**diopathic
- **S**arcoidosis
- **C**onnective tissue disease

- **O**ccupational exposure
- **A**llergic reaction
- **I**nfection
- **R**adiation.

INFLUENZA INFECTION: CLINICAL MANIFESTATIONS

Her Child's Sickness Made Child's Mother Frustrated And Needy

- **H**eadache
- **C**hills
- **S**ore throat
- **M**alaise
- **C**ough
- **M**yalgias
- **F**ever
- **A**norexia
- **N**asal congestion.

KLEBSIELLA: DETAILS

FUN PASs

- **F**at capsule
- **U**rinary tract infection (UTI)
- **N**onmotile
- **P**neumonia
- **A**lcoholic
- **S**epsis.

PULMONARY EMBOLISM: RISK FACTORS

ROM IS PERFECT

- **R**est (bed-ridden)
- **O**besity
- **M**alignancy
- **I**mmobilization
- **S**urgery
- **P**regnancy
- **E**lderly
- **R**oad trip

- **F**racture
- **E**strogen (postpartum)
- **C**ardiac disease
- **T**rauma.

PULMONARY FIBROSIS: DIFFERENTIAL OF BOTH UPPER AND LOWER LOBES

CARS ARE BeST

Lower lobe:

- **C**ryptogenic fibrosing alveolitis
- **A**sbestosis
- **R**adiation
- **S**ystemic sclerosis

Upper lobe:

- **A**nkylosing spondylitis
- **R**adiation
- **E**xtrinsic allergic alveolitis
- **Be**ryliosis
- **S**arcoidosis
- **T**uberculosis (TB).

PNEUMOTHORAX: PRESENTATION

HOT CRAP

- **H**yperresonance
- **O**nset sudden
- **T**rachea deviation
- **C**ollapse seen in X-ray
- **R**educed breath sounds (and dyspnea)
- **A**bsent fremitus
- **P**leuritic pain.

RESPIRATORY DISTRESS SYNDROME IN INFANTS: MAJOR RISK FACTORS

Children's Distress Problem

- **C**esarean section
- **D**iabetic mother
- **P**rematurity.

Reproductive System

CHAPTER

10

ENDOMETRIAL CARCINOMA: RISK FACTORS

ME, HE, DON

- **M**enstrual irregularity
- **E**strogen therapy
- **H**ypertension
- **E**lderly
- **D**iabetes
- **O**besity
- **N**ulliparity.

ENDOMETRIAL CARCINOMA: RISK FACTORS

ENDO HAs risk factors

- **E**lderly
- **N**ulliparity

- **D**iabetes
- **O**besity
- **H**ypertension
- **A**ge (increased).

GYNECOMASTIA: CAUSES

DALS

- **D**igitalis
- **A**lcohol
- **L**eydig cell tumors
- **S**ertoli cell tumors.

OVARIAN CANCERS: IMPORTANT TYPES BY WHO CLASSIFICATION

She May Be Experiencing Cancer Knowingly Found in Sweet Girls Of The D Enclave

Surface:

- **S**erous
- **M**ucinous

- **B**renner
- **E**ndometrioid
- **C**lear

Metastatic:

- **K**rukenberg

Sex cord:

- **F**ibroma
- **S**ertoli-Leydig
- **G**ranulosa-theca

Germ cell:

- **O**varian choriocarcinoma
- **T**eratoma
- **D**ysgerminoma
- **E**ndometrial sinus.

POLYCYSTIC OVARIAN DISEASE: CLINICAL FEATURES

OO! HI!

- **O**ligomenorrhea
- **O**besity

- **H**irsutism
- **I**nfertility.

SCROTUM MASSES

EH! TV IS HOT

- **E**pidymal cyst
- **H**ydrocele
- **T**umor
- **V**aricocele
- **I**ndirect inguinal hernia
- **S**permatocele
- **H**ematocele
- **O**rchitis
- **T**orsion.

CHAPTER 11

Skeletal System

CARCINOMAS HAVING TENDENCY TO METASTASIZE TO BONE

The Pure Love Kicks Badly

- **T**hyroid
- **P**rostate
- **L**ung
- **K**idney
- **B**reast.

MARBLE BONE DISEASE: SIGNS AND SYMPTOMS

MSC BLADE

- **M**ultiple fractures
- **S**plenomegaly

- **C**ranial nerves restricted
- **B**lind
- **L**iver enlarged
- **A**nemia
- **D**eaf
- **E**rlenmeyer flask deformity.

OSTEOMYELITIS: COMPLICATIONS

BRIEFS

- **B**acteremi/Brodie abscess
- **R**eactive amyloidosis
- **I**ntraosseous (Brodie) abscesses
- **E**ndocarditis
- **F**ractures
- **S**quamous cell carcinoma/Sinus tracts.

RHEUMATOID ARTHRITIS: FEATURES

HE IS THE MAD RAMBO

- **H**uman leukocyte antigen-DR (HLA-DR4)
- **E**rythrocyte sedimentation rate **(**ESR) increase

- **I**nflammatory synovial tissue/Idiopathic
- **S**mall joints affected in starting
- **T**-cells (CD4)/TNF
- **H**uman leukocyte antigen-DW (HLA-DW4).
- **E**xtra-articular features (restrictive lung disease, subcutaneous nodules)
- **M**orning stiffness
- **A**nkylosis/Atlantoaxial joint subluxation
- **D**eformities
- **R**agocytes/Rheumatoid factor (anti-IgG)
- **A**utoimmune
- **M**etacarpophalangeal (MCP) joints stiff and affected
- **B**ilateral
- **O**steopenia.

CHAPTER 12

Miscellaneous

CAPSULATED BACTERIA

FAKE MBBS HaS Panicked Your Profession

- *Francisella*
- Anthrax (*Bacillus anthracis*)
- ***K**lebsiella*
- ***E**. coli*
- **M**enigitidis (*Neisseria menigitidis*)
- ***B**acteroides*
- ***B**rucella*
- ***S**treptococcus pneumoniae*
- ***H**aemophilus influenzae*
- ***S**almonella*
- ***P**asteurella*

- *Yersinia pestis*
- *Pseudomonas.*

COMMON COLD: VIRAL CAUSES

RIMPA

- **R**hinoviruses
- **I**nfluenza viruses
- **M**yxoviruses
- **P**aramyxoviruses
- **A**denoviruses.

FRAGILE-X SYNDROME: FEATURES

$CAM_{(4)}$ EL

- **C**hromosome staining discontinued
- **A**nticipation shown
- **M**ale more affected
- **M**ental retardation (2nd most common genetic cause)

- **M**acrognathia
- **M**acroorchidism
- **E**verted eyes
- **L**ong face with large jaw.

NECROSIS: THE FOUR TYPES

God Can Create Life

- **G**angrene
- **C**aseous
- **C**oagulation
- **L**iquefactive.

RNA VIRUSES: NEGATIVE STRANDED

PARO's Boy Friend

- **P**aramyxo
- **A**rena
- **R**habdo
- **O**rthomyxo

- Bunya
- Filo.

RNA VIRUSES: POSITIVE STRANDED

They Can Concentrate Regularly For Positive Response

- Toga
- Corona
- Calici
- Retro
- Flavi
- Picorna
- Reo.

RNA ENVELOPED VIRUSES

Finally CAB Reached FORT Properly

- Flavivirus
- Corona

- **A**rena
- **B**unya
- **R**habdo
- **F**ilo
- **O**rthomyxo
- **R**etro
- **T**oga
- **P**aramyxo.

STAPHYLOCOCCUS AUREUS: DISEASES CAUSED

FAST SPIN

- **F**ood poisoning
- **A**cute endocarditis
- **S**kin infections
- **T**oxic shock syndrome
- **S**epsis
- **P**neumonia
- **I**nfective arthritis
- **N**ecrotizing fasciitis.

STREPTOCOCCUS PYOGENES: DISEASES CAUSED

LESS PC IN MP

- **L**ymphangitis
- **E**rysipelas
- **S**carlet fever
- **S**treptococcal TSS
- **P**haryngitis
- **C**ellulitis
- **I**mpetigo
- **N**ecrotizing fasciitis
- **M**yositis
- **P**neumonia.

STREPTOCOCCUS PYOGENES: VIRULENCE FACTORS

SMS HEAD

- **S**treptolysins
- **M**-protein

- **S**treptokinase
- **H**yaluronidase
- **E**xotoxin
- **A**nti-C5a peptidase
- **D**NAses.

TURNER SYNDROME: COMPONENTS

LUNCH

- **L**ymphoedema
- **U**nderdeveloped ovaries (causing sterility, amenorrhea)
- **N**eck webbed
- **C**ardiac abnormalities (specifically coartication)
- **H**aving widely spaced nipples.

UREASE: POSITIVE ORGANISMS

PHUNC

- ***P**roteus* (leads to alkaline urine)
- ***H**elicobacter pylori*

- *Ureaplasma* (renal calculi)
- *Nocardia*
- *Cryptoccocus* (the fungus).

WHIPPLE'S DISEASE: FULL FEATURES

HIP PILLS

- **H**yperpigmentation of skin
- **I**nvolvement enteric
- **P**AS positive granules in macrophage
- **P**olyarthritis
- **I**nfection with *Tropheryma whippelii*
- **L**ymphadenopathy
- **L**oss of weight
- **S**teatorrhea.

Index

A

Abdominal pain 26
Abscess 54
  in crypts 7
Accumulated
  glycogen 45
Acidity 5
Acne 23
Activated protein C 11
Acute
  endocarditis 70
  pancreatitis 53
  post-streptococcal
glomerulonephritis 31
  tubular necrosis 35
Addison disease 22, 24
Adenomatous polyps 1, 2
Adenoviruses 67
Adherin pili 30
Adrenal cortex 25
Adrenal of medulla 26
Adrenocorticotropic
  hormone 22
Agglutination 41
AIDS pathogens 38
Akinesia 49
Alcohol 5, 17, 32, 41, 60
Alimentary system 1
Alkaline urine 72
Allergic reaction 55
Alzheimer's disease 47
Amenorrhea 72
Ammonium magnesium
  phosphate 31
Anaplastic carcinoma 28
Anemia 4, 12, 16, 20, 64
Aneurysm 9, 17, 18

Angiotensin-converting enzyme inhibitors 6
Ankylosing spondylitis 57
Ankylosis 65
Anorexia 55
Anterograde amnesia 52
Anthrax 66
Antiphospholipid antibody 12
Antitoxin 46
Anxiety 27
Aorta coarctation 14
Argyll-Robertson pupils 50
Arrhythmia 15, 17, 18, 33
Arteriovenous fistula 9, 34
Asbestosis 57
Ascaris lumbricoides 4
Aspartate transaminase 18
Aspergillus 39
Aspiration 53
Aspirin 5
Asteroid bodies 43
Asthmatic wheezing 2
Ataxia 50, 51
Atelectasis 54
Atherosclerosis 8, 36
Atlantoaxial joint subluxation 65
Attack of acute gouty arthritis 32
Autoimmune 22

B

Bacillus
anthracis 66
cereus 3
Bacteroides 66
Bad oral hygiene 5
Bat-wing lung X-ray 14
Beryliosis 57
Bloated face 31
Blood pressure 10

Bone alterations 36
Breast 63
Brodie abscess 64
Bronchial obstruction 54
Bronchiectasis 54
Brucella 66
Buerger's disease 9

C

Calcium 31
Calculi 31
Cancer 48
Candida albicans 38
Capillary
  microaneurysm 9, 34
Capsulated bacteria 66
Carcinoid syndrome 1
Carcinoma 7
Cardiac
  abnormalities 72
  disease 57
Cardiomyopathy 43
Cardiopulmonary 36
Cardiovascular system 8
Catalase positive
  organisms 39
Catecholamine
  secreting 49
CD4 helper cells 43
Cellulitis 71
Cerebral
  cortex atrophy 47
  fat pads 23
Cesarean section 58
Charcot joints 50
Chest pain 10, 19
Chills 55
Chorioretinitis 51
Chromosome staining
  discontinued 67
Chronic
  liver disease 17
  ulceration 10
  ulcerative colitis 1
Cirrhosis 17
  and chronic liver
    disease 17

Clostridium
botulinum 3
perfringens 3
Coke-colored urine 31
Collagen fiber
weakness 23
Colon
cancer 2
carcinoma 1
Comedones 23
Common cold 67
Confusion 51
Congenital infection 51
Congestive
cardiac failure 17
heart failure 36
Conjunctivitis 16
Connective tissue
disease 54
Coronavirus 42
Cough 55
C-protein deficiency 11
Cramps 33
Creatine kinase-MB
isoenzyme 18
Cryptococcus
neoformans 38
Cryptogenic fibrosing
alveolitis 57
Cryptosporidium
parvum 38
Cushing's
syndrome 14, 23
Cutaneous flushing 1
Cystine 31
Cytomegalovirus 38
Cytopenias 40

D

Dandy-Walker
syndrome 47
Deep venous
thrombosis 11
Deficiency of muscle
phosphorylase 45
Deformities 65

Diabetes 59, 60
- insipidus 43
- mellitus 9, 11

Diaphoresis 26
Diarrhea 2
Diet and lifestyle 15
Diffuse
- intravascular
  - coagulation 35
- lung infection 53

Digitalis 60
Digoxin toxicity 33
Dilated superficial
- veins 11

Disseminated
- intravascular
  - coagulation 39

Doppler ultrasound 11
Dorsal column
- degeneration 50

Down's syndrome 47
Dressler's syndrome 17
Drowning 53
Dryness of
- lips and month 16
- palms and soles 16

Dysgerminoma 61
Dyspnea 44

E

Echovirus 42
Eczema 44
Edema 4, 34, 40
Electrolyte imbalance 36
Elevated
- cholesterol 8
- creatine kinase 45
- erythrocyte
  - sedimentation rate 12
- vitamin D value 44

Emphysema 54
Encephalitis 51
Endocarditis
- 12, 13, 16, 64

Endocrine system 22

Endometrial
  carcinoma 59
  sinus 61
Endometrioid 61
Endothelial cells 40
Enterobacter cloacae 37
Enterobius
  vermicularis 4
Enterococcus faecalis 37
Enterovirus 42
Enzyme
  deficiencies 15, 24
Epidymal cyst 62
Erlenmeyer flask
  deformity 64
Erysipelas 71
Erythema
  nodosum 43
  of palms, soles 16
Erythroblastosis
  fetalis 15
Erythrocyte
  sedimentation rate 64
Erythromycin 6
Erythropoietin 35
Escherichia
  coli 2, 3, 37, 50
Estrogen 6, 57
  therapy 59
Ethacrynic acid 6
Exercise 11
Exotoxin 30, 72
Extrinsic allergic
  alveolitis 57
Eye dysfunction 21

F

Facial edema 31
Fat
  capsule 56
  embolism 14
  in urine/sputum 14
Fatigability 27
Fatty liver 4
Fever 20, 42, 55
Fibroma 61

Flavivirus 69
Folate deficiency 17
Follicular carcinoma 28
Food poisoning 3, 70
Fractures 14, 64
Fragile-X syndrome 67
Francisella 66
Furosemide 6

G

Gangrene 9, 68
Gastrointestinal
  disturbances 36
Glance on very
  important urinary
    disease 35
Glomerular disease 35
Glucose intolerance 23
Goiter 23, 28
Gout 32
Granular mucosa 7
Growth retardation 23
Gynecomastia 60

H

Haemophilus
  influenzae 40, 50, 66
Hashimoto's disease 24
Head trauma 48
Headache 26, 55
Heat
  intolerance 28
  stable 40
Helicobacter pylori 72
Hemanigoblastomas 21
Hematocele 62
Hematuria 12, 32
Hemolysis 41
Hemolytic anemia 15
Hemorrhagic gastritis 36
Hepatic
  encephalopathy 33
Hepatitis A 42
Hereditary
  sperocytosis 15
Hirsutism 23, 62
Homocystinemia 10

Hormones 29
Human
  leukocyte antigen 65
  papilloma virus 5
Hyaluronidase 72
Hydrocele 62
Hyperaldosteronism 14
Hypercalcemia 25
Hypercortisolism 23
Hyperglycemia 23
Hyperkalemia 36
Hyperpigmentation
  of skin 73
Hyperresonance 58
Hypersplenism 40
Hypertension 8, 14, 16, 23, 36, 59, 60
Hyperthyroidism 27
Hypokalemia 33
Hyponatremia 22
Hypotension 22
Hypothyroidism 24
Hypotonia 33

I

Idiopathic
  polymorphic rash 16
IgA nephropathy 34
Immune mediated
  noncaseating
    granulomas 43
  inflammation 2
Immunohemolytics 15
Impetigo 71
Increased
  coagulability 21
  jugular venous
    pressure 19
Indirect inguinal
  hernia 62
Ineffective antimicrobial
  therapy 13
Infarctions 17
Infection 12, 15, 35, 48, 55
Infectious-subacute
  thyroiditis 24

Infective arthritis 70
Infertility 62
Inflammatory synovial tissue 64
Influenza
- infection 55
- viruses 67

Influenzae 48
Inguinal hernia 62
Integumentary system 29
Intermittent claudication 10
Interstitial lung
- disease 54
- fibrosis 43

Intraosseous abscesses 64
Iodine deficiency 24
Iron
- deficiency 41
- containing lesions 30

J

Jugular venous pressure 19

K

Kawasaki disease 16
Kidney 63
- cysts 21

Klebsiella 37, 56, 66
Korsakoff's psychosis 52
Kwashiorkor 4

L

Lactate dehydrogenase 18
Large intestine 6
Left ventricular failure 18
Leprosy 29
Leukocytopenia 12
Leukocytosis 12

Leukoplakia 5
Leydig cell tumors 60
Lipid pneumonia 54
Liver 21
 disease 41
Long face with
 large jaw 68
Loss of weight 73
Low fiber, high fat diet 2
Lower lobe 57
Lung disease 43
Lymphadenopathy 73
Lymphangitis 71
Lymphatic system 38
Lymphoadenopathy 16
Lymphoedema 72

M

Macrocytic anemia 17
Macrocytosis 41
Macrognathia 68
Macroorchidism 68
Malabsorption 4
Malaise 55
Marasmus 4
Marble bone disease 63
McArdle's syndrome 45
Medullary thyroid
 carcinoma 26, 28
Menigitidis 66
Meningcoccus
 disseminated
 intravascular
 coagulation 22
Meningitis 48
Menstrual irregularity 59
Mental retardation 67
Metabolic acidosis 36
Metacarpophalangeal
 joints 65
Microangiopathic
 hemolytic anemia 42
Microcytic anemia 41
Morning stiffness 65
Multiple
 endocrine neoplasia
 5, 25, 26
 fractures 63

Mural endocarditis 12
Muscular
  system 45
  weakness 27
Myalgias 55
Mycobacterium
  avium intracellulare 38
  leprae 29
Myelodysplasia 41
Myocardial
  infarction 17, 18
  rupture 18
Myocarditis 51
Myoglobinuria 45
Myositis 71
Myxedema coma 24
Myxoviruses 67

N

Nasal congestion 55
Necrosis 68
Necrotizing fasciitis 70, 71
Neisseria meningitis 50
Nelson's syndrome 22
Nematodes 4
Neoplasm 32
Nephritic syndrome 34
Nephronal disease 32
Nephrotic syndrome 33
Nervous system 47
Neuroblastoma 49
Neurologic
  dysfunction 20
Neuroma 26
Neutrophil
  chemotaxis 39
  invasion 7
Night attacks 32
Nitric oxide 39
Nocardia 73
Noniatrogenic
  neoplasms 23

Noninfectious
endocarditis 13
Nonsteroidal anti-
inflammatory drugs 6
Nulliparity 59

O

O-antigen 39
Obesity 10, 56, 59,
60, 61
Obligate intracellular
organisms 13
Occupational
exposure 55
Ocular lesions 43
Oligomenorrhea 61
Onset of puberty 23
Ophthalmoplegia 51
Orchitis 62
Osteomalacia 36
Osteomyelitis 64
Osteopathy 43
Osteopenia 65
Osteoporosis 36
Otitis 48
Ovarian
cancers 60
choriocarcinoma 61

P

Palpitations 26, 27
Pancreas 21
Pancreatitis 6
Papillary
carcinoma 28
muscle 17
Paralysis 30
Parameningeal
infection 48
Paramyxoviruses 67
Parathyroid 25
Paroxysmal
nocturnal
hemoglobinuria 15
rise in blood pressure
26

Pasteurella 66
Penicillamine 6
Peptic
  ulcer 5
    disease 36
  ulceration 25
Pericarditis 17-19, 36
Pharyngitis 71
Pheochromocytoma 14, 21, 26
Phlebitis 10
Picorna viridae 42
Platelet count low 20
Pleural adhesions 54
Pleuritic pain 58
Pleuritis 54
Plummer-Vinson syndrome 5
Pneumocystis carinii 38
Pneumonia 56, 70, 71
Pneumothorax 58
Poliovirus 42
Polyarthritis 73
Polycystic ovarian disease 61
Polyposis 1
Polyuria 33
Port-wine stains 21
Prematurity 58
Propagation 20
Prostate 63
Prosthetic valve endocarditis 13
Protein S and protein C 19
Proteinuria 12, 33
Proteus mirabilis 37
Pseudomonas 39, 67
  aeroginosa 30, 37
Pseudopolyps 7
Pulmonary
  embolism 56
  fibrosis 57
  system 53
Pulsus paradoxus 19
Pyogenic meningitis 50
Pyruvate kinase 15

R

Radiation 53, 55, 57
Rapidly progressive glomerulonephritis 34
Ratio of animal fat 1
Raynaud's phenomenon 9
Reactive amyloidosis 64
Recessive inheritance 45
Red blood cell trauma 15
Reduced breath sounds 58
Refractory congestive heart failure 14
Remnants of old ulcers 7
Renal
  calculi 43, 73
  failure 21, 35, 42
Reproductive system 59
Resection of mycotic aneurysm 13
Respiratory distress syndrome in infants 58
Restrictive lung disease 65
Reticulocytes 41
Reticulocytosis 17
Retrograde amnesia 52
Rheumatic heart disease 16
Rheumatoid arthritis 64
Rhinoviruses 42, 67
RNA viruses 68, 69

S

Salmonella 3, 66
Sarcoidosis 22, 54, 57
Scarlet fever 71
Schaumann calcifications 43
Scrotum masses 62
Sensory loss in affected skin 30
Sepsis 53, 56, 70
Serratia marcescens 37
Sertoli cell tumors 60
Seventh cranial nerves palsy 43

Shock 53
Shooting pain 50
Sickle cell 15
Silent thyroiditis 24
Sinus tracts 64
Sinusitis 48
Skeletal
  muscle only 45
  system 63
Skin infections 70
Slow growing fastidious organisms 13
Sodium loss 36
Sore throat 31, 55
Spermatocele 62
Splenectomy 48
Splenomegaly 40, 63
S-protein deficiency 11
Squamous cell carcinoma 64
Staphlococcal infections 44
Staphylococcus
  aureus 3, 39, 70
  saprophyticus 37
Steatorrhea 73
Stenosis of renal arteries 14
Steroids 6
Stone 25, 32
Stooped posture 49
Streptococcus
  pneumoniae 40, 48, 50, 66
  pyogenes 71
Streptokinase 72
Streptolysins 71
Strong family history of colon cancer 1
Subacute
  right-sided
    endocarditis 13
  thyroiditis 24
Subcutaneous nodules 43, 65

Superficial nodular 10
Sweating 27
Syphilis 50
Systemic
  lupus
    erythematosus 34
  sclerosis 57

T

Tabes dorsalis 50
Tamponade 17
T-cell suppression 38
Teratoma 61
Tetanus 46
Tetany 33
Thalassemia 15, 41
Thiazides 6
Thrombocytopenia 12, 20, 42, 44
Thromboembolic disorders 17
Thrombosing vasculitis 10
Thrombotic
  thrombocytopenic
    purpura 20
Thrombus 19
Thyroid 25, 63
  carcinoma 28
  disease 17
  storm 27
Thyroiditis 23, 24
Thyrotoxicosis 16, 23
  syndrome 27
Torsion 62
Toxic
  megacolon 7
  shock syndrome 70
Toxoid 44
Toxoplasma gondii 38, 51
Trachea deviation 58

Tracheostomy 46
Trauma 27, 57
Traveller's diarrhea 3
Tremor 28
Trichuris trichiura 4
Triglycerdides and fats 8
Tropheryma whippelii 73
Troponin 18
Tuberculosis 22, 38, 57
Tubulointerstitial
  nephritis 35
Tumor 62
  necrosis factor 39
Turner syndrome 72

U

Ulcerative colitis 2, 6
Ulcers 6
Ureaplasma 73
Urethritis 32
Uric acid 31
Urinary
  free corisol and
    glucose 23
  obstruction 35
  system 31
  tract infection
    30, 37, 56
Urine pleomorphic
  microvilli 27

V

Vaccines 44
Varicocele 62
Vascular
  insufficiency 22
  obstruction 35
  trauma 21
Vasculitis 16
Venography 11
Vermis small 47

Vibrio
parahaemolyticus 3
vulnificus 3
Virchow's triad 21
von Hippel-Lindau 21

W

Water on brain 47
Weakness of muscles 33
Weight loss with good appetite 28
Wernicke-Korsakoff's psychosis 51
Whipple's disease 73
Wiskott-Aldrich syndrome 44

Y

Yersinia pestis 67